BeauTEAful Skin

By:

Laura Victoria

Contents

CHAPTER ONE

Everybody Loves Tea

As a matter of fact, there are many kinds of tea that you could find in the market such as green tea or herbal tea. People use these different types of tea regularly since tea has always been known for its positive effects on humans that it is even referred to by the easterners as the key to wisdom and happiness. Tea is well known for its huge nutritional value for ages. Among these types of tea comes white tea. Most of us know the value of other teas, but have you ever thought of using white tea instead?

White tea is considered the highest of all tea types in nutritional value. White tea contains very useful elements and is also very rich in antioxidants, but the question is, "how is white tea manufactured?" White tea is obtained from the leaflets of the tea plant, these leaflets then get steamed to get white tea and surprisingly it keeps its values when steamed, white tea is subjected to the minimum amount of treatment that's why it is the most expensive among the other types of tea.

Several studies have been carried out regarding this topic and they all assured the extreme benefits of white tea. Due to these benefits, it came to be considered as a better and healthier alternative to coffee, which contains a high percentage of caffeine. White tea is more beneficial than black teas or even green tea. Black and green teas have almost equal benefits, but white tea comes first when it comes to benefits. The reason behind that is the less processing that white tea undergoes compared to the other types and this helps in retaining a high level of phytochemicals. Furthermore, white tea does not require much time or labor to be produced as that required for black or green tea due to its less processing. Besides, it protects the body from the occurrence of some diseases due to its various nutrients as well as its antimicrobial properties.

History of the White Tea

It is believed that white tea was firstly originated in China. In 1700, the modern process of white tea production emerged. With time, various kinds of white tea were exported from China to the rest of the world. The types of white tea vary according to the type of tea bushes that it is produced from.

White tea may mean a type of the different type of tea, which normally has either a young or minimally a kind of processed leaves from the plant of Camellia Sinensis. There is no globally recognized definition of what white tea should be and it has little agreement from international bodies. According to some, white tea is a type of tea that is normally dried and has no additional processing done to it. To others, white tea refers to it as one that has tea buds and young leaves, which have been fired prior to drying or steamed. But most definition does agree to this, nevertheless, white tea is neither oxidized nor rolled, giving rise to a flavor that is characterized to be lighter when compared to green or traditional black teas. It is primarily harvested in China in the Fujian Province. Recently, it is produced in Taiwan, Eastern Nepal, India and Galle (Southern Sri Lanka). The source of white tea is from the buds and the leaves that weren't matured. Before the buds open finally, they are picked. The buds and leaves are not left to dry or wither in natural sun. So why is it called "White Tea"? The name is gotten its appearance, it has fine silvery white hairs on the buds that haven't been open from the tea plant, and this makes the plant to have a whitish appearance. Do you know it has beverage? Yes! The color is not colorless or white but has a pale yellow and light to the taste.

Composition of the White Tea

Just like green and black tea, white tea is gotten from the Camellia sinensis plant and this has polyphenols. The health effects of the white tea are produced because of the presence of a set of phytonutrients. There is a different amount of catechins and polyphenols for each white tea. The concentration of some white tea is the same as green teas. This can account for the different diversity of the tea plant from the tea itself was picked, the way it was processed and the cultivation technique used.

Manufacturing of White Tea

The manufacturing of white tea follows a simple process and it is as follows:

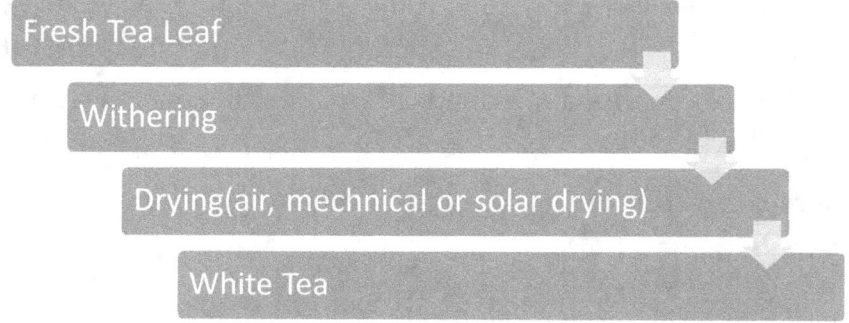

Fresh Tea Leaf

Withering

Drying(air, mechnical or solar drying)

White Tea

White tea is among the category of teas that don't require shaking, rolling or panning. The choice of raw material that is used in the manufacturing of white tea is tremendously stringent; all that is needed is the plucking of the leaves of the young tea that has fine hair and this can give you a good worth of white tea of a high pekoe value

Type of White Tea

Just like other tea types, white tea also has it varieties that give the drinkers the choice to choose the type they want. Knowing the difference between each type of white tea can be a daunting task. The white tea does have different names and varieties, but the name doesn't give an insight into what the tea is all about. That is why we ensure in researching to let you know of the different type of white tea. So what are they?

White Tea Types

The different varieties of white tea can be distinguished on quite a number of factors, which includes the origin and the ingredient that is added to the leave such as fruit. Listed below and explained are some of the popular varieties of white tea.

- **Silver Needle** – After water tea, this is the most sought after. This variety of white tea is harvested in early spring right before the tea bus has transformed into leaves. At this point, handpicking is the best option for the bud and this should be dry and warm. The mild and sweet flavor of this variety of white tea is what has given it a wide recognition among other types of white tea.

- Long Life Eyebrow – this variety of white tea is regarded to be the least among the types of white tea such as White Peony and Silver Needle. In terms of appearance, it is darker and has much richer flavor when you compare it to other varieties of white tea.

- Tribute Eyebrow – Just as the Long Life Eyebrow is lesser, so is the Tribute Eyebrow. It is normally harvested after White Peony and Silver Needle. Tribute Eyebrow is handled somewhat inversely and has more of a darker appearance and is like the Long Life Eyebrow.

- White Peony – In terms of quality, this is the second after Silver Needle. The White peony is reaped when there are two leaves and a bud. Cool-wise, it is darker and has a stronger taste than the Silver Needle.

- Snowbud – This is not the favorite among the four different varieties of white tea. This is reaped only when there are leaves and buds. It has a clear color and mild flavor when compared with all the other varieties of white tea.

In as much as there are different varieties of white tea, it's left for you to experience the taste for yourself. White tea is really hard to come by in the market. The drinking of the white tea is better than taking a bitter medicine. White tea is ideal for your health and has a lot of benefits. This shouldn't be taken by you allow, initiate your family members in taking white tea every day to release stress and have a good body system

White Tea vs. Green Tea

Have you thought about a single plant producing two different types of tea? The green tea and the white tea all proceed from the same source, the Camellia Sinensis. The white tea leaves are the first to be reaped before the green tea leaves. They have a lower caffeine level and antioxidant. This has made the green tea to be even more popular. We are talking about white tea, but why is it that green tea is more popular and the white tea is unknown? This is simply because the white team is very rare to see and reaped during the early spring. Even when you find it, it is very expensive. The benefit of green tea and white tea are almost the same since they have the same antioxidants and nutrients. But the white tea is much better than the green tea in every area of comparison. This following are some of the key reasons why you should consider taking more of the white tea.

- **Caffeine**

They both contain a lower level of caffeine than all other types of teas, but the content of the caffeine in the white tea is lower to the green tea. When serving, the white tea has about 5mg lower content of caffeine. If you want to relax at night, white tea is the best option.

- **Antioxidants**

By now you already know that antioxidants aid in the fighting of free radicals in the body that fight your cells and cause diverse kind of diseases and speed up the aging processing you. The white tea leaves are reaped when the leaves are very young. The buds have much antioxidant content when compared to other type of tea. The white antioxidant in the white tea makes it the best for tea drinkers.

- **Taste**

The primary reason must people drink tea is because of the taste. The taste may be different for each person, most people find a sweet and mild taste much better and white tea has more appealing taste than green tea. Looking for a tea with a lower caffeine content and smooth taste then the white tea is your best option.

Proper Brewing of White Tea

For most individuals, the intake of white tea is something that is an experience. For others, the overall process right from the picking process to the washing, they are seen as a ritual. White tea is a delicate kind of tea and properly care throughout the process. In the brewing of the white tea, the most important thing is to make sure that it still retains all the good flavor and antioxidants.

Store Your Tea

In the process, the first step is the brewing of the white tea to make it the perfect tea. If not properly stored, the white tea will virtually lose it antioxidants and nutrients. The white tea should be kept in a container that is tight and away from heat, light, and moisture. If it is not properly stored, the tea will lose its great taste that you so much desired.

The Process of Brewing the White Tea

There are different steps involved in the process of brewing the white. The brewing should be done rightly to ensure that you will get the finest taste each time. The rushing of the process of brewing the white tea will cause you to lose its healthy antioxidants and flavor. The following are the steps for the brewing.

Step 1: Water: The enemies of the white tea is hot water and hard water and affects it very much. To get the best cup from the white tea, you should verify that the water isn't hard or have much minerals. Investing in a water filter should be a top priority if you want to get the best from the white tea. Alternatively, you can purchase water from stores. It's essential that during the process of brewing the white tea, the water shouldn't be too hot. After the water is boiled, allow it to cool for some minutes. If the water is much hotter, you will not enjoy the benefit of the antioxidants contained in the white tea.

Step 2: Tea: the quantity of the tea you use is more of a personal choice. For you to derive the ideal result, you should use the complete leaves. Irrespective of the part you are using, either the tea bag or the leaves, it is very essential, more usage of the white tea will give you a stronger taste.

Step 3: Steeping:- During the brewing process of the white tea, it should be properly steeped. Steeping has to do with the placing of the tea bag or tea leaves into the water for it to bring out the nutrients and flavor into the water. The perfect timing is essential in the steeping process, a minute is perfect. Once you have steeped the tea, you don't need to discard the leaves immediately. They can be used more often, but the only thing is that as you use it frequently, you lose the flavor that it has.

Looking for a Healthier You?

The mildness of the white tea is what many people love. It relieves stress when you take a sip after a long day. It hasn't come to the notice of many how best it is for them to drink the white tea. The White tea antioxidants level is higher when compared to other tea products. I know you don't know, so let me inform you, white tea contains antiviral and antibacterial effects that support your body in fighting against some infections as well as helping your dental health. Choose white tea for a better health regimen daily

Antioxidants in White Tea

Do you know what the antioxidant does in white tea? I can bet you don't. Well, the antioxidant high content known as epigallocatechin gallate fights the free radicals in your body. Free radicals also fight the cells that are in your body and kill off things that could speed up the aging process and cause disease. The following are some of the diseases that free radicals may result to:

- Diabetes
- Heart disease
- Stroke
- Cancer

There are many problems it can cause, but these are just a few of them.

CHAPTER TWO

Health Benefits of White Tea

Researchers have conducted a lab experiment by putting a human cell in a container and applied some white tea on it, they observed a notable decrease in fat level in the same cell. Therefore, white tea extract prevents obesity cells that contribute to the formation of fatty tissues of the body of completeness, also it helps in burning cells, which had just formed, increases the metabolism process which results in slimming.

A recent British scientific study revealed that white tea has many health benefits, and this is because it contains high levels of antioxidants that may protect against cancer and heart diseases, outperforming the 21 different species of plants and aromatic herbs. Professor Declan Naughton, a specialist in inflammatory diseases of the joints at the University of "Kingston" in London, said that white tea helps in the fight against the manifestations of aging and contains high levels of antioxidants that may protect against rheumatoid arthritis. It is the properties of white tea that help to reduce weight, inhibits the multiplication of cancer cells and also limits at the same time the formation of new cells. The effectiveness of the white tea is evident in the treatment of cutaneous radiation injury cases. Let's discuss each benefit in detail:

Antioxidant and Anti-Aging Properties

White tea helps you maintain a good, youthful health state and that is due to its anti-aging and antioxidant properties.

Our bodies contain some free radicals and those radicals help in damaging many of our organs, including our skin. And hence, they contribute to the overall aging process of our skin. Now you might be wondering, how is white tea helpful regarding my skin? White tea neutralizes those radicals and thus reduces their destructive effects on your body. Many studies suggest that white tea increases the effects of antioxidants of plasma as well as most of our organs. Those studies also mentioned how white tea and its extracts help in cell neuroprotection due to their antioxidant properties. In addition to this, those antioxidants present in white tea help in reducing the risk of early aging.

Healthy and Youthful Skin

Moreover, white tea helps you to have a healthy skin, as it has some protection abilities that protect you from the harmful effects that UV light could have on your skin. Due to the previously mentioned antioxidant properties that white tea possesses, it helps in the recovery of damaged skin. Moreover, It helps in killing bacteria and prevents the possibility of acne. It helps in keeping the skin in a good condition which is another function for the antioxidants. In addition to all that, it prolongs aging symptoms as well, it helps reducing skin wrinkling, dark spots in skin as it usually prevents the enzymes that reduce collagen and elastin, it reduces the probability of knees and elbows inflammation. It improves the digestion process and prevents stomach ulcers.

Oral Health

One of the various benefits of white tea is the improvement in oral health. Due to the presence of some contents such as tannins in white tea helps in preventing the growth of bacteria causing plaque formation. In addition to this, fluoride found in white tea helps in reducing the risk of cavities and tooth decay. White tea was also found to prevent teeth inflammation since it cleans the mouth from bacteria and harmful cells. It doesn't cause coloring of the teeth as coffee or black tea.

Effects On Diabetes

Diabetic people find white tea very beneficial to them as it relieves some of their illness symptoms such as their excessive thirst, their increased secretion of insulin and it also decreases the plasma glucose levels.

Cancer Prevention

White tea contains the polyphenol that enhances the immune system and protects the body against cancer. It can reduce or even eliminate the risk of cancer. The same as green tea, white tea is beneficial in preventing many forms of cancer, for instance, lung cancer. Researchers suggest that white tea has the potential of becoming a chemopreventive, anticancer agent. Regarding white tea and its extracts, they may offer great help in preventing new cell growth. However, further research must be carried out in order to confirm if white tea truly has anticancer properties for other cancer types as well as lung cancer.

Cardiovascular Disorder

In addition to this, white tea puts the risk of any cardiovascular disorders to a minimum. Due to the presence of flavonoids in white tea, which might also be found in some vegetables and fruits, the risk of cardiovascular orders is decreased. Moreover, those flavonoids also help in the improvement of dyslipidemia as well as decreasing blood pressure. White tea also helps in reducing the harmful cholesterol LDL in the blood. A study found that white tea is used to have the ability to prevent bad gene mutation in the body cells. It also helps in preventing deep vein thrombosis as it improves the blood circulation.

Antibacterial Properties

White tea has some antibacterial properties that can protect your body from many infections that cause bacteria and other microorganisms. Bacterial attacks of the immune system are some of the main causes that result in some medical conditions and diseases. However, white tea with its antibacterial properties can protect you from bacteria as well as other germs. White tea is also used as a key ingredient in many of the cleansing products that we use daily, such as hand or facial soap. Furthermore, the intake of white tea may provide relief from common cold and flu to those who suffer from such symptoms.

The Benefits of White Tea in Weight Loss

White tea has been utilized in 2010 at a lot of western countries, it usually contains a lot fewer calories than the other types of tea. A lot of people take it regularly in order to help them in their struggle of losing weight. Wrong food choices, as well as bad habits, may result in a gradual but enormous weight gain. Sometimes, shaking that extra gained weight is no easy task, especially if you don't have enough time to be working out. In this case, a diet plan might seem as the closest option, but we all know that sticking to a strict diet is not as easy as it sounds and for some might be even brutal. If you are one of the many people struggling with weight loss, here is a surprise for you.

White tea is considered very valuable to those who aim at weight loss, studies have shown that white tea prevents the formation of new fat cells known as lard cells, it also helps in reducing the amount of fat in the body and burning those cells to get effective weight reduction.

White tea has a notable amount of caffeine that also helps in reducing the amount of fat, it helps in increasing the benefit of dietary fibers when processed inside the human body, not convinced yet, ok. Don't take it as an assignment to drink a cup of white tea today or anything but apart from this, white tea has a smooth taste as well, you can add sugar, milk but you are adding more calories this way, so take care.

White tea also helps in reducing the feeling of hunger, so you eat less and in turn lose some pounds.

White Tea- Selection and Consumption Tips

It is better to consume white tea, brewed in the form of loose leaves. Consumption of white tea in this form guarantees the existence of nutrients in their actual primitive form. This is way better than consuming it in the form of tea bags since tea bags definitely need more processing procedures to be produced.

How can white tea be brewed? You might ask; brewing of all types of tea is almost the same. It is better for you to use clean and pure water while brewing and also the water should be heated enough but not boiled so as not to destroy the sensitive components of your tea. If you favor a more concentrated taste, you might steep your tea for a couple of minutes or add an extra amount of tea leaves above the average which is about one to two spoons of white tea per cup.

If you really want to benefit from your white tea consumption, your daily intake should be about two to four cups. You can even use the brewed tea leaves more than once, it might also be beneficial since it gives you a chance to extract all of the nutrients within your tea leaves. One thing you need to care of, in the case of brewing more than once, leave your tea for longer than the first time. FYI, its preferred not to have it before going to bed, try having it 15 minutes after a meal. Furthermore, you can try different flavors of tea available in the market and determine your favorite. Increase your daily intake of white tea, hence increase your health.

When can it be harmful?

White tea can cause anemia as it prevents the body from absorbing the useful minerals as iron and calcium from food which can later cause insomnia, having white tea in the early morning can affect your health badly, it can help in the formation of a delicate membrane on the inside walls of your stomach which can decrease the amount of gastric juice and leads to digestion problems, so as you see here, timing can completely invert the benefit to a harm.

White tea facial skin home recipes

Facial steam

Steam must be one of the essential parts of your facial skin routine since it opens and cleans the pores, softens the skin and improves the blood circulation in your face. Plus, the process is very relaxing.

Ingredients:

- White tea, mint, rosemary and rose water.

How to prepare:

Step 1: In a pot, boil a liter of water.

Step 2: Place the ingredients in a heat-safe, large bowl and pour the water over them and leave them to steep for a minute or so.

Step 3: Place your face above the bowl, about 12 inches away from the steam and don't forget to cover your hair with a towel. Before doing so, you need to make sure that the water did cool down a bit so as not to get burnt. Remain in front of the steam for a minute, take a break then repeat.

Step 4: After you complete your facial steam, apply a nourishing moisturizer on your face.

It is recommended to repeat the whole steam process more than once a week for better skin results.

The White Mask

Ingredients:

- One spoon of full cream yogurt
- White tea packet

Preparation:

In a clean bowl, mix a large spoon of the full cream yogurt with the contents of the tea packet, then start mixing them properly. We then leave the mixture about half an hour before we apply it to our faces. Leave it for 15 to 20 minutes and then wash your face with water, you will notice the refreshment instantly.

The mask is usually called a refreshment mask because of its effect of making people active and refreshed afterward as well as of its effect in lightening the skin. It is usually recommended to make the white tea mask after steaming and cleaning your face. The mask is suitable for every skin type there is.

The Remedy for Better Looking Eyes

Ingredients:

- White tea

Procedures:

Take two teaspoons of white tea and add some water. Heat them all together until boiling. After that let it cool down for a couple of minutes before you steep the tea. Once the tea reaches a temperature that you can handle to put on your face, soak a piece of cotton in the liquid and place it on your eyes. The heat will cause your pores to open up which will allow the tea to penetrate your skin. It will remove any swallowing or tiredness from your eyes, leaving them looking fresh and bright due to the presence of both antioxidants and caffeine.

Facial Mask for Dry Skin

Ingredients:

- White Tea, Honey & Ginger

Preparation:

Take a teaspoon of white tea and boil it with half a glass of clean water. Leave it until it is warm then add the honey and ginger to it and stir. Apply the mixture on your skin and leave it for fifteen minutes. Rinse off with lukewarm water and gently dry. This mask works perfectly against acne and skin renewal.

White Tea with Facial Cleanser

Ingredients:

- White tea and your own facial cleanser

Procedures:

Add white tea to your daily cleanser by soaking the tea bag into super-hot water, empty the contents in a cup then add your cleanser. The cleanser and the tea will blend together. Use a spoon to mix them together well and apply on your skin. Go prepare your breakfast or tidy your bed until the time passes, then rinse it off. Do that in the morning before heading to work, it will leave your skin looking amazing.

White tea toner

Ingredients:

- White tea and rose water.

Procedures:

Put the rose water in a pot. Heat it gradually until boiling. Place it in another heat resistant cup and before it starts to cool down, place a bag of white tea in the cup. Leave them for three to five minutes in order to infuse, then throw the tea bag out. Place the liquid in a spray bottle or if you prefer a regular bottle and put it in a fridge. Apply it on your face at night as a toner. Keep repeating that every day before going to bed. With time, it will tighten your skin, cover any wrinkles if there are and make you look younger. You can even use it in the morning, directly after walking up and washing your face. It will make your face look revived and if you concentrated on applying it under the eyes, it will make you look more awake due to the effect of caffeine.

No Hassle Recipes

1. Whenever you are drinking tea, after you finish your cup, take the tea bag out, cut it open and empty its contents in the cup. Add some honey to turn it into a paste and apply to your skin. Leave it for about ten minutes, then rinse it off with cool water.

2. Prepare yourself a cup of green tea and leave it to cool. Instead of drinking it after that, go straight to the sink and put some tea in your hands and splash it on your face. Keep doing so until your cup is empty, then rinse off with cool, clean water.

3. If you have a date or some big event and you want to look nice and fresh but do not have enough time for a full facial, here is a trick. Take a white tea bag and soak it in super-hot water. Squeeze it a bit and run it over your face, then rinse off. This will leave your face glowing and relaxed.

4. **Tea Toner:** Make a pot of tea and leave it to cool. Get a piece of cotton and dip it into the tea. Rub the cotton piece all over your face, preferably twice a day. Don't forget to always keep it in a cool place till it runs out.

Bottom Line for White Tea

The drinking of the white tea is better than taking a bitter medicine. White tea is ideal for your health and has a lot of benefits. This shouldn't be taken by you allow, initiate your family members in taking white tea every day to release stress and have a good body system

Here you have it, the many benefits of white tea and even some facial tricks to help you look your best. Hope you found it interesting. Don't forget, never slip on your white tea.

CHAPTER THREE

Green Tea: Nature's Panacea to Many Health Challenges

The health benefits of Green Tea are immense. Any time you take a sip of green tea, remember that you are gulping one of the healthiest beverages on earth. There have been in-depth research into the vast subject of alternative medicine over the last few decades and these studies have led to large scale discoveries on the health-boosting properties of certain plants. These discoveries are not entirely new because, for many centuries, traditional healers in different parts of the world had used herbs to tackle several diseases that plagued the human body. However, research and empirical evidence have given credibility to these healing methods and have validated the postulation that certain plants contain properties that provide immune support to the body, helping the body rid itself of materials that are harmful to it.

One of those super healthy plants is Green Tea. This is not to say that Green Tea and indeed any other nutrient-rich plant should become a substitute for proper medical diagnosis and treatment of diseases. When there is significant proof of the onset of a disease, you should seek proper medical attention from professionals rather than resort to self-help through the intake of concoctions. The risks of self-help to the body are numerous. In the first instance, treatment is administered after proper diagnosis has been done and the cause of the health challenge established. If you opt for self-treatment, you stand the risk of taking the wrong medication because what you thought was a particular ailment may be something else after all.

Apart from the need for medical diagnosis, there is also the need for proper dosage prescriptions. You stand a very high chance of filling up your system with too much of a particular substance present in one of these so-called super foods. This can be counter-productive, creating deeper problems for the body than what you set out to cure. So, patient analysis and proper dosage prescriptions belong to the realm of the professionals and you should make it a point to contact them when a particular disease sets in.

Nevertheless, health-boosting foods like Green Tea are great for preventive care. The old saying that 'prevention is better than cure' is very apt. Green Tea contains antioxidants that help the body dispense with toxins that are harmful to it, thereby preventing any disease that such toxins would have caused. This and many more health properties of Green Tea will be covered in detail in this book.

Background Information about Green Tea

Green Tea is made from leaves called Camellia Sinensis. There are several varieties of Green Tea, depending on the type Camellia Sinensis that is used to make the tea, the cultivating method, production process and time of harvest.

Steeping refers to the process of making a cup of tea for consumption. It tells you the quantity of water you need for a certain amount of tea. So don't run away to fill up the flask just yet! You should take Green Tea in measured quantities. That is what steeping or brewing is all about. Typically, two grams of tea per 100ml of water should be fine. You can translate that to about one teaspoon of Green Tea per 150ml cup of water.

Another component of the steeping process is the ideal temperature levels you need to achieve to get the best out of your Green Tea. This is never cast in stone. You do not need to walk around with a thermometer to check how hot the water is before adding your tea. The temperature level differs with each type of tea. Anything from 61 to 87 degrees Celsius should be alright. Brewing time can also be a factor in the mix to achieve healthy levels of the tea. The usual time ranges from thirty seconds to three minutes. What you should pay attention to and avoid is making your tea too hot and keeping it for too long. When Green Tea is overheated, it becomes very bitter. This is due to the release of excessive amounts of a compound known as Tannins. Some people prefer to leave the tea in the pot and to continuously add hot water for drinking until the flavor completely fades away.

The Origins of Green Tea

From available records, Green Tea originated from China before its production spread to other countries and regions of Asia. A book on traditional Chinese medicine written over one thousand years ago chronicled the use of Green in traditional medicine. Subsequent authors also listed the health benefits of the Green Tea in relation to the human vital organs. They also provided information on the various brewing styles of Green Tea. Green Tea was used in ancient China for the treatment of headaches and depression. It was quite effective at the time and became really popular among the people of China and the rest of Asia.

In contemporary times, the use of Green Tea has become common and acceptable in many countries in the world. The consumption of the tea gathers momentum each passing day as researchers reel out the results of their studies on Green Tea. People all across the world now utilize Green Tea mainly for its health benefits and its flavor.

The Nutritional Content of Green Tea

Green Tea as earlier noted is one of the richest types of teas available. The list below shows clearly the nutritional component of Green Tea:

Green Tea Composition

S/N	Compound	Percentage
1	Catechins	30 - 42
2	Flavonols	5 - 10
3	Other Flavonoids	2 - 4
4	Theogallin	2 - 3
5	Other Depsides	1
6	Ascorbic Acid	1 - 2
7	Gallic Acid	0.5
8	Quinic Acid	2
9	Other Organic Acids	4 - 5
10	Theanine	4 - 6
11	Other Amino Acids	4 - 6
12	Methylxanthines	7 - 9
13	Carbohydrates	10 - 15
14	Minerals	6 - 8
15	Volatiles	0.02

Credit: http://www.greenteanutritionfacts.com/

Green Tea Nutritional Facts

S/N	Nutrient	Amount Per Serving – 100ml
1	Calories	2
2	Sodium	3mg
3	Potassium	27mg
4	Total Carbohydrate	0.2g
5	Protein	0.2g
6	Vitamin C	6mg
7	Calcium	3mg

S/N	Nutrient	Amount Per Serving – 100ml
8	Iron	0.2mg
9	Riboflavin (B2)	0.05mg
10	Niacin (B3)	0.2mg
11	Vitamin B6	0.01mg
12	Magnesium	2mg
13	Panthothenic Acid	0.04mg
14	Copper	0.01mg
15	Manganese	0.31mg

Credit: http://www.greenteanutritionfacts.com/

CHAPTER FOUR

The General Health Benefits of Green Tea

G reen Tea is a nutrient-rich herb. Over the years, the health benefits of the compounds contained in Green Tea have been established. However, clinical research does not show enough supporting evidence to this. A report published by a panel of scientists in 2011 suggested that the claims of the health benefits of Green Tea were not supported by sufficient scientific evidence.

Nevertheless, researches conducted on the various compounds contained in Green Tea have proven a direct linkage between the components of the tea and relief from health issues. Nutritionists like Beth Reardon in Boston have identified the Catechin content of Green Tea as its biggest health benefit. He noted (to the excitement of Green Tea lovers) that catechins are antioxidants that fight and in some instances prevent cell damage. And since Green Tea does not pass through rigorous processing methods before consumption, the Catechin content remains intact as you pour the content into your cup.

How about improved blood flow and lowering of cholesterol? You have every reason to jubilate if you have challenges in the line of blood flow and cholesterol. In 2013, a review of many studies on Green Tea was done and what was discovered was amazing. Green tea can help you prevent a range of heart-related issues from high blood pressure to congestive heart failure. In one of the studies carried out in Switzerland, MRI scans revealed that people who drank Green Tea regularly had more activity going on in the working memory area of their brains. So diverse research works have laid credence to the fact that Green Tea is beneficial to human health. We will open your eyes to the general health benefits of Green Tea in the following part of this book.

1. Healthy Teeth and Gums

One of the benefits of consuming Green Tea is that it will promote your oral health. In 2009, a study was published in the Journal of Periodontology found that regular consumption of Green Tea reduced symptoms of periodontal disease. This was linked to the Catechin content. Catechins are known to reduce inflammations in the body and thus were found to help the body combat the inflammatory tendencies of periodontal bacteria. Catechins ability to tackle bacteria and to reduce acidity in the saliva and plaque in the teeth makes it ideal for combating many variations of oral health issues. If you are drinking Green Tea regularly, you can be sure that bad breath will not be part of what you worry about when in the midst of people. However, be sure not to add any sweetener to your cup of Green Tea if you intend to enjoy the full benefits in your mouth.

2. Weight Loss

Weight loss is one benefit of Green Tea that users allude to globally. Clinical studies suggest that Green Tea helps to boost metabolism in the body and helps to burn fat. Furthermore, the Catechins in Green Tea is known to produce thermogenesis which is a known help in weight loss. Green Tea has proven a useful resource for obese people or those who are slightly overweight, helping them lose and maintain healthy weights. However, to have Green Tea help you combat weight effectively, you would need to take up to three cups every day. For the weight loss enthusiast or those on a strict weight loss regime owing to ill-health, when next you return from the road walk, have a cup of Green Tea instead of some sweetened fruit juice. Repeat this two more times in a day and you are on your way to a healthy weight.

3. Lowers Cholesterol

Green Tea helps with improved performance of the heart immensely. This it does by reducing the total bad (LDL) cholesterol in the system while raising the good cholesterol or HDL. A research work based on the study of a population revealed that men who drank Green Tea regularly had lower cholesterol levels than those who did not drink Green Tea at all. Another research in 2011 published in the American Journal of Clinical Nutrition showed that consuming Green Tea significantly reduced total serum cholesterol and LDL across 14 random trials conducted on 1100 persons. A study done on animals also showed that polyphenols present in Green Tea have the capacity to prevent cholesterol from being absorbed by the intestines and to help the body speed up the emission of cholesterol. It is the powerful anti-oxidant - Epigallocatechin Gallate (EGCG) content in Green Tea that helps the body to achieve this. Rather than choke the body with those unhealthy snacks and sugary drinks that do more damage to the body, make do with five cups of Green Tea every day and get the biggest reduction in cholesterol.

4. Helps Regulate Blood Sugar and Provides Succour for Diabetes

Green Tea has been one of the ways that people over the years have controlled blood sugar. Studies have linked drinking Green Tea with prevention of the development of Type 1 Diabetes and slowing down its progression in the event that it had developed. Diabetes is a disease related to insulin deficiency in the body whereby the body's ability to regulate blood glucose is severely hampered. Green Tea helps to regulate the glucose levels in the blood. Research has been conducted which points to the fact that regular consumption of Green Tea can help you effectively manage Type 2 Diabetes.

5. Improves Eyesight

If you are seeking ways to boost your eyesight, then there is great news for you. The well-known anti-oxidant in Green Tea called Catechins is known to be able to penetrate the tissues of the eyes. When it does this, it triggers anti-oxidant activity in the eyes, helping the eyes get rid of harmful toxins. A publication in the Experimental Eye Research Journal in 2001 showed that Green Tea could actually prevent blindness induced by cataract. The researchers showed that the part of the eyes that retains the highest amount of absorbed catechins was the retina, with the cornea retaining the lowest. This went to show that the antioxidant in Green Tea can serve as a protective mechanism for the eyes.

6. Soothes Ear Infection

Your ear can respond to the antioxidant in Green Tea too. Practice has proven that people with ear infections only need to dip a cotton ball in Green Tea until it is soaked up by the liquid and then use it to clean the affected ear. This helps to reduce and subsequently eliminate the infection.

7. Eliminates Allergies

The EGCG content of Green Tea is a known and proven anti-allergy compound. Another compound in Green Tea, Polyphenols has been validated by a study published in the Journal Cytotechnology as capable of reducing pollen allergies. Furthermore, Quercetin, a flavanol in tea possesses the ability to alleviate a histamine response. This portends that it provides the body with the necessary capacity to fight the allergy. Do you have allergies? Green Tea may just be your best bet to curb that.

8. Alleviates Liver Problems

A population-based research discovered that men who consumed more than 10 cups of Green Tea per day were least likely going to develop liver disease. Apart from this, Green Tea also showed the capacity to protect the liver from the damaging effects of harmful toxins and compounds like alcohol. Catechins in Green Tea have the potential of treating a viral inflammation of the liver known as Hepatitis. Drinking 10 cups of bitter Green Tea is not what you would ordinarily prefer right? The immune benefits that come with the consumption of this liquid are massive. Just that drinking up to ten cups in a day may not be a very good option because of the caffeine content of Green Tea which may prove an overdose in this case. You don't want your concentration to be hampered when driving after a consistent gulping of Green Tea.

9. Cold and Flu

You know how uncomfortable these two can make you be, don't you? Tackle them effectively with few cups of Green Tea and the Vitamin C content of the green liquid will help your body to send them packing. Not only will Vitamin C help eliminate cold and flu, it can also help the body prevent them from setting in at all.

10. Tackles Many Types of Cancer

By far one of the most potent activities of Green Tea in the body is its fight against the several types of cancer. The strongest antioxidant in Green Tea – EGCG is a known destroyer of cancer cells through the destruction of the cells' mitochondria. There is more good news here; Green Tea will not leave you with any of the side effects that the conventional treatment methods like chemotherapy would bring. This postulation is backed by research published in the journal called Molecular Nutrition and Food Research. A top expert and associate professor of Food Science at Pennsylvania State University corroborated this report by pointing out that EGCG causes the formation of reactive oxygen species found in cancer cells and this essentially damages mitochondria in the cells thus making the mitochondria produce more reactive oxygen species. With time, the mitochondria will lose its defensive mechanisms and succumb to the anti-oxidant genes. In this weakened state, cancer cells surrender to EGCG and are eliminated.

Several population-based studies have confirmed the potency of Green Tea for the prevention and treatment of several types of cancer. For instance, it was observed that a country like Japan where the consumption of Green Tea is very high has relatively low levels of cancer prevalence. Clinical studies also suggest that the polyphenols in Green Tea may be able to help people prevent cancer and some even link it with the death of cancer cells. Polyphenols have also been known to prevent cancer cells from growing.

The following types of cancer have been known to succumb to the potency of the antioxidants in Green Tea: bladder, oral, breast, ovarian, colorectal, esophageal, lung, pancreatic, prostate, skin and stomach cancers. The antioxidant and alkaline properties of Green Tea make it a potent force against cancer. However, some studies have also cautioned that the research backing up the potency of Green Tea against cancer cells have not been exhaustive.

11. Inflammatory Bowel Disease (IBD)

If Green Tea can help you deal with colorectal or colon cancer, then it sure can help the body dispense with inflammatory bowel disease because anyone stricken with the latter stands a high risk of the former. Green Tea battles the two types of inflammatory bowel disease, namely; the Crohn disease and ulcerative colitis. It does this by reducing the inflammation usually associated with the two diseases.

12. Helps Combat Depression and Stress

From historical times, Green Tea was used to combat depression and stress. This is because it contains the amino acid – Theanine which provides a calming and tranquilizing effect when absorbed by the body. It's soothing sensation helps a depressed or deeply stressed person to sleep. With time, barring the elimination of some remote causes of depression like a failed relationship or the pain of losing a loved one, Green Tea would cure depression and help the body to be relieved of stress.

13. Lowers Blood Pressure

Taking up to five cups of Green Tea in a day will help to lower blood pressure, studies show. One of such studies, published in the British Journal of Nutrition in October 2014 disclosed that long-term intake of Green Tea can help reduce blood pressure significantly. In a test case, after 12 weeks of drinking Green Tea, blood pressure became lower by 2.6mmHg systolic and 2.2 mmHg diastolic. Reducing systolic blood pressure to this extent would expectedly bring the risk of stroke by eight percent and the risk of coronary artery disease death by up to five percent. If you have a raised blood pressure, the best bet is not to worry and complicate the situation, start enjoying Green Tea today in addition to other core lifestyle changes and such a health condition will become a thing of the past.

14. Enhances Bone Health

The anti-oxidant and anti-inflammatory properties in Green Tea can help check bone loss and could help the body produce bone-building cells.

15. Helps to Prevent Parkinson's and Alzheimer's Diseases

Green Tea helps with the repair of damaged cells in the brain and further protects brain cells from dying thus eliminating to an extent the risk of brain disorders. Green Tea has been known to be effective in treating Parkinson's disease and Alzheimer's disease.

The Unusual Things about Green Tea

There are many things that make Green Tea unusual. From its very unusual discovery mythology to the way it is consumed in many places, Green Tea has some unusual dimensions.

- Legendary accounts have it that the Chinese Emperor Shen Nung discovered Green Tea when leaves blew into his pot of boiling water.

- China is known to be the birthplace of tea.

- There are over 1500 species of tea, amongst all of these; Green Tea is one of the most potent in terms of health benefits.

- Coming next to water, tea is the most-consumed drink in the world. Who knows? Probably that is why more and more health benefits of Green Tea are being discovered.

- Green Tea can be used to cook. Apart from being consumed as a drink, Green Tea has a very strong flavor that is used as a seasoning for food. You may want to test this one after all the health benefits would still be intact.

- Green Tea can be used to eliminate refrigerator odor. So you can wrap them in a thin cloth bag today and place in the refrigerator for a few hours and watch how they make your refrigerator odour-free.

Chapter Five

Green Tea and Skincare

One thing you should add to your beach pack the next time you are heading to the beach for a day out should be a packet of Green Tea. In addition to your sunscreen and sunglasses, your Green Tea will help to protect your skin from the damaging consequences of the ultraviolet rays of the sun.

The much-talked-about Catechins will do some superb work in enhancing your skin's resistance to the ultraviolet rays of the sun, reducing the likelihood of premature aging. Are you worried about the redness of the skin after a day out in the sun? Green Tea is naturally poised to protect your skin from this. The British Journal of Nutrition published a study done in the Year 2013 showing that a relatively low dosage of (just over 500 mg) Green Tea each day in addition to 50mg of Vitamin C taken for 12 weeks can remarkably reduce the consequence of ultraviolet radiation on the skin.

The study discovered that Green Tea worked in this direction by reducing the effect of inflammation produced by exposure to ultraviolet radiation. This study revealed something novel; the first time it was determined that oral doses of Green Tea could find their way to the tissues of the skin to work against the damaging properties of the sun's ultraviolet radiation.

The anti-oxidant properties of Green Tea have consistently shown the possibility of slowing down the onset of aging and getting rid of wrinkles. The antioxidant, EGCG prevents the activation of collagen-digesting enzymes known as matrix metalloproteinase. These are the enzymes responsible for the wrinkles found on the human skin. By rubbing Green Tea extracts directly on the skin as a lotion or drinking the right dosage of the liquid, you can actually take advantage of the anti-oxidant properties of Green Tea to stop premature aging or wrinkles from setting in.

How Green Tea is used for Skincare

As earlier discussed, Green Tea's antioxidants have untold benefits for the human skin. The tea can be used for the treatment of many skin conditions and more importantly to retain a glowing skin texture. The following are some of the ways that Green Tea can be used for skincare.

1. Acne Treatment

The anti-oxidant, anti-inflammatory and anti-bacterial properties in Green Tea make it the ideal herb to effectively combat acne. Bear in mind that Green Tea also has some anti-fungal properties which would defeat the growth of fungi infections on the skin. It has been scientifically proven that Green Tea reduces the production of sebum by 50 percent and its anti-bacterial properties help to destroy the bacteria that cause acne. To treat acne with Green Tea, there are two steps, namely:

- Purchase a moisturizer or lotion with Green Tea extract and rub on the acne-stricken face regularly

- Prepare a natural Green Tea extract and simply rub it on your face and body regularly. Allow them to remain on the skin for some time before rinsing.

- Drink four to five cups of Green Tea daily to reduce hormonal acne.

2. Improving Skin Complexion

Green Tea helps to improve skin complexion as well. The anti-oxidant properties help to flush out toxins from the skin, heal scars and remove blemishes. Green Tea also helps to reduce the possibility of any inflammation on the skin. The Medical College of Georgia corroborated this in a research work by showing that Green Tea helps in the rejuvenation of the skin.

To get the best out of Green Tea facial treatment for complexion and skin rejuvenation, you can follow the simple steps below:

- Empty the content of two green tea bags into a cup

- Add between one and two teaspoonfuls of raw honey

- Mix a little quantity of lemon juice

- Apply the mixture on the face and allow to remain for up to ten minutes

- Rinse off with lukewarm water

- Repeat this every day for two to three weeks

3. Do away with Puffy Eyes and Dark Circles on the Face

The compound called Tannin in Green Tea helps to get rid of puffy eyes and dark circles on the face. This it does by shrinking the blood vessels underneath the skin of the eyes, helping it reduce swelling and puffiness. The Vitamin K content of Green Tea also helps to treat the dark circles that appear on the skin of the face. In attempting to treat puffy eyes and dark circles, the following steps should be followed:

- Put two used green tea bags in a refrigerator for up the thirty minutes

- Remove them and place on your closed eyelids and relax for up to 15 minutes

- Apply this remedy two times every day until your desired results are achieved.

4. Do away with Aging on the Skin

Green Tea has proven anti-aging properties embedded in its anti-oxidants and this help to delay the onset of aging on the skin. Some of the signs of aging on the skin are sagging, age spots, fine lines, and wrinkles. The polyphenols contained in Green Tea help to neutralize harmful free radicals on the skin. These free radicals if left unchecked can cause severe damage to the skin. The neutralization of free radicals on the skin also helps to check and prevent skin cancer. To tackle aging and its attendant effects on the skin with Green Tea, the following simple steps should be adhered to:

- Mix one tablespoonful of Green Tea with three tablespoons of yogurt
- Add a little quantity of turmeric powder
- Rub this mixture on your face and around your neck
- Allow it to remain on your skin for at least 20 minutes.
- Rinse with lukewarm water
- Repeat process once or twice every week for best results

5. Tone the Skin

Green Tea is very effective in serving as a natural toner for the skin. It helps to draw out toxins and impurities, reduce large pores, and keep the skin hydrated. This gives the skin both a healthy and a glowing look. To achieve this, the following should be done:

- Brew at least two cups of Green Tea
- Allow it some minutes to cool
- Add a few drops of essential oil (any type you feel comfortable with) to it
- Put this liquid in a spray bottle
- Spray on your face or apply to your face using a cotton ball at least two times daily to get the best results

Steaming the Face

A great way of treating facial conditions, drawing out toxins, debris, dirt, and impurities is by having a facial steam. This can be done through the following steps:

- Boil water and pour out into a bowl
- Take a green tea bag, cut it and empty its content into the water
- Allow this to brew and cool for five minutes
- Drape a clean towel over your head and bend over the bowl
- Your face should be about 30 centimeters away from the bowl to be able to trap the steam
- Stay in that position for about five minutes

Creating Your Own Tea Face Mask

You can use the Green Tea face mask to treat and manage any of the facial conditions explored earlier. From the treatment of acne to managing wrinkles and aging, Green Tea is effective in making the face smooth. Using a bag of Green Tea, you can create your own face mask and allow Green Tea detoxify your skin and eliminate the free radicals that are causing you problems.

These are the steps you need to follow to create your own unique Green Tea face mask.

1. The Simple Tea and Rice Flour Mask
    - Brew a pot of tea and allow it to cool

- Mix three tablespoons of cool tea with three to four tablespoons of rice flour
- Wash your face with a cleanser and dry with a clean towel
- Apply the mixture as mask to your face
- Leave it for 15 minutes
- Rinse it off with lots of water

2. Green Tea Oats and Egg Face Mask

- Empty the content of three green tea bags into a bowl
- Add a small quantity of facial moisturizer into the bowl
- Add granulated sugar or sea salt to the bowl
- Add two egg yolks
- Add a small amount of water
- Add a small amount of oats
- Mix all these ingredients together, adding either water or oats until the desired texture is achieved.
- Apply the mask to your face
- Leave it on your face for minutes
- Wash the mask off with water

3. Green Tea, Honey and Oatmeal Face Mask

- Boil water and dip a green tea bag in it

- Squeeze out the liquid to the bowl and allow it to cool.

- Boil some more water to steam your face

- After ten minutes, scrub your face

- Mix the vitamin C powder, honey, and oatmeal

- Apply the paste to your face and neck

- Leave the mask on your face for between one to three hours

- Wash off with water

Face Washing Techniques

Washing your face may not be as easy as it sounds. There is an art to it if it has to be done properly. Here are three techniques:

1. Wash your face with lukewarm water and with a cream cleanser. After washing, use a towel to dab your face dry. Do not rub so you don't stretch your skin and cause wrinkles

2. Dip a cotton ball in a toner and swipe it around your face targeting the areas on your face where there are problems. One soaked cotton ball is enough to achieve this

3. Wet your face with lukewarm water and use your fingertips to apply your cleanser. Your fingertips are the best to use for this as sponges or washcloths can irritate the skin.

Bottom line for Green Tea

Green Tea has been used for its health value from centuries ago. Up till now, the tea is still being used to treat or manage many diseases. However, you need to know how to apply your Green Tea Remedy for best results.

CHAPTER SIX

What about Oolong Tea?

O olong tea originates from China and is essentially transcribed from two basic words which mean "Dragon" and "Black" in English. Apart from its deeper meaning, both words that for the Oolong in English practically make a description of the shape of the oolong leaves in its original state. The Oolong tea goes through a process of distinct semi-oxidization which scope covers about 1 to 99 percent. Immediately the picking of the tea is done with, the leaf withers and is semi-oxidized in the sun and the shade gets dried up. Once this is completed, they are tossed into a basket in order to break down the cells that are on the top of the leaves. This stops the process of oxidization. Various methods are used during its production stage. The heating methods include the perfect roasting of the tea leaves in a number of steps which normally occurred all through the night. The Oolongs are most times processed through a wood or charcoal which gives rise to a special and unique flavor to the diverse finishing styles. In conclusion, the leaves are rolled or curled into a crispy shape, which has the resemblance of a tiny black dragon, therefore this is the reason behind the description of its name. They are usually harvested late in the spring when compared to white teas or green tea and are more mature. White tea or green teas are usually harvested late April or early May. The manufacturing of the oolong tea is kind of complicated because some steps are repeated different times before the final browning a bruising of the leaves is gotten. Withering, firing, shaping and rolling are similar to the black tea, but the only difference is that much temperature and attention to accurate timing is required or necessary

Brief History of Oolong Tea

The tea was nicknamed to the creator of the oolong tea. It is a tea from China that has distinctive and unique characteristics and is mainly produced in Guangdong and Fujian, as well as Taiwan. The most famous teas from Chinese include Dahongpao, Iron Lohan, Phoenix Bush, Phoenix Narcissus, Tieguanyin and White Crest, the most known Taiwanese Oolong's tea include Wenshan, Dongding, and Oriental beauty. The Taiwanese Oriental Beauty is widely known as Formosa Tea or due to the abundance of white pekoe, it is also called White Tipped Oolong Tea. The ambassador from England to China gave some Oolong tea to the Queen of England in early 19th Century. The uniqueness of the aroma and taste made the queen to have a keen interest in it. That wasn't all that made the queen to love it, its appearance is another feature and this was different to any kind of tea she has seen in England before. Then as a result of this, she gave it the name "Oriental Beauty". As a tea that is slightly oxidized, it has an aroma and taste that is between black teas and green teas. The different kind of Oolong tea has a different array that is like the green tea or almost like the black tea. But this is dependent on the degree of oxidation while carrying out the processing

Oolong's Predecessor - Beiyuan Tea

The life span of the oolong tea dates back to the Fujian Province, this history goes back as over a 1000 years to a traditional kind of tea that is known as Beiyuan Tea. The Beiyuan tea was the foremost tribute tea that is known. A tribute tea is a kind of tea that is given in tribute to the royal family or emperor and produced in Fujian. During the Song Dynasty period, it was among the most well-known teas that were produced. The Phoenix Mountain region in Fujian is where the Beiyuan is located and has been in the production of tea right before the Tang Dynasty. The type of tea was a compressed one with leaves that are compressed into cakes. The tea lost its uniqueness with the royalty and this gave rise to the production of a partially oxidized leaf tea rather than the authentic oolong tea.

The Legendary Story of Oolong Tea

There is a different story about the source of the Oolong. In the times of the Qing dynasty, in Fujian, a tea farmer was picking up tea on a particular day from far he saw a deer. After deciding to kill it rather than finishing the picking of the tea. He couldn't finish with the picking and it was on the next day he finally finished. The edges of the leaves had moderately oxidized and it brought in a good and surprising aroma. After he finished the process of picking it, he became surprised as to find a totally new strong sweet flavor. This didn't have any form of bitterness to it, which was normally produced in the previous form. This person decided to give it the name "oolong" and the tea was named to the guy. His actual name was Wu Liang.

The History of Taiwanese Oolong Tea

During the early 1800s, a tea merchant from Fujian collected some seeds to Taiwan for him to see how the plants will grow there. This was like an experiment, but his outcome was very successful and in the next year, there has been a widespread production of tea in Tea. Nevertheless, most of the tea in the first half of the century were returned back to Fujian, for it to be processed there instead of Taiwan. In 1868, everything changed when John Dodd, a British decided that it was enormously inefficient. This made him seek the services of tea masters in Fujian to start the processing of the tea in Taipail. This was very successful and in the next year, he made a shipment of about 127 tonnes of the tea. In the United State, it was called Formosa Tea and became successful there too. Right from that time, the oolong tea became one of the most globally transported type of tea from Taiwan.

Production of Oolong Tea

Oolong Tea has 7 processing steps before you can get all the nutrients from the leaves. The following are the steps:

1. **Withering**

This is the first step in the processing of the oolong tea. Firstly, the leaves that were picked are spread out. Do you know how to spread it out? It's simple, inside and/or outside in the sun. This is done to make the cell walls of the leaves to be soft. This process sucks out the moisture in the leave to the top to undergo evaporation, makes the leaves not to be stiff and starts the natural enzymatic fermentation process. After this is done, it is ready to undergo the next stage of its processing. One importance of this stage is it, it reduces the taste of the tea leaves from being grassy.

2. **Tossing/Bruising (Turning Over)**

This is simply known in Chinese as "Shaking". This name came because, in the olden days, the leaves were merely shaken off into a wicker basket. Nowadays, this process is done with the help of a specially designed machine to break down the leaves further through a mechanical process. In the first step (Withering), the breaking down is done by a chemical means. Why go through this stress? It improves the oxidation and combines the chemical elements with the leaves from the stem. This balances the flavor and removes its bitterness nature of the tea.

3. Oxidization (Partial and Full)

The process that is used in the Black and oolongs tea continues its nature procedure of fermenting through by letting the leaves to rest after the tossing/bruising or withering steps. The amount of fermentation in the oolong tea that is made will be determined by the time that is allocated to it. During this stage, the leaves turn to a red color or darker green, this is because of the breaking down process of the cell structure of the leaves. It's flowery, grassy and fruity taste features start to develop at this stage

4. "Kill-Green" (also known as Fixing")

At this stage, the growing processes and natural fermentation are stopped within the leaves and without any damage to them. Hand pressing the leaves in a hot pan, steaming it and baking methods are used. After this stage comes the next step, which is the Rolling or forming of leaves.

5. Rolling/Forming

The leaves that go through the cold and/or hot rollers begin to break down the leaves slightly. This intensifies the flavor of the tea and establishes its shape.

6. Drying

At this stage, it creates a final damp content of the leaves and the fermentation process is stopped. It also prevents the growth of mold, develops the aroma of the tea and finally removes any grassy taste of the leaf.

7. **Firing**

It has different methods of being roasted in a basket or in a pan with electric heat or charcoal and gives off a smoky flavor or fruity feature. Whatever method that is more comfortable with you, should be strictly adhered to.

So when it has to do with the processing of the oolong tea, the steps are very similar and overlapping with one another. Nevertheless, the oolong tea has a very special category, this is as a result of the roasting/baking technology that is applied. The importance of this process in the processing of the oolong tea cannot be overemphasized because it has an effect on the final taste, appearance, and aroma of the oolong tea. This is one of the reasons in this book we have dedicated to giving the way it is produced.

The Purpose or Effects of the Roasting Oolong Tea

1. **Reduce Water Content:** The Roasting of the oolong tea will help in the reduction of the capacity of water in the oolong tea. When the water content in the Oolong tea is between 4 to 6 percent, this can stop the deterioration of the tea and gives it a prolonged storage life.

2. **Remove Raw Smell:** The second reason for the removal of the raw smell from the tea is by dehydrating or heating, the sugars and amino acids

that are in the leaves and this will be converted into chemical components, which will produce a more pleasant and richer smell when the leaves are soaked.

3. **Stop Oxidation**: Finally, it stops the process of the oxidation of leaves and gives room for the tea to be in perfect shape for more ripening if it is properly stored. Proper storage is necessary.

Control Factors & Considerations of Oolong Tea

Water content

The major significance of the roasting of the oolong leaves is to reduce the content of water in the tea leaves to 4 to 6 percent and at the end slow down the oxidation of the leaves. This procedure makes the storage of the tea to stay longer. The different water content in tea leaves has their own divers roasting conditions. No much high-tech tools are used for measuring. The judge of the final outcome is the tea master and this is based on the experience of the quantity of the water content that is still left in the tea. Mold will appear in a situation where the water is above 8.8 percent, but immediately it is above 12 percent, then deterioration will gradually take place in the tea leaves. Normally, teas with a high content of water, the temperature for roasting must be between 95 °C and 100 °C. If peradventure, the process of roasting takes more than three hours, then the temperature has to be reduced 85 °C or so. The reducing of the temperature makes it bring forth the niceness and rich aroma of the tea. This is not the only factor that the tea master considers, there are also others which are discussed below. The tea leaves that have a high content of water must be spread out sparingly, else the leaves will have an effect as a result of inappropriate exposure to air and the quality of the tea will be compromised.

Tenderness of raw tea leaves

Roasting older and thicker tea leaves needs a medium temperature of about 85 to 90°C while the time range for roasting is between 4 to 10 hours and this is dependent on the different kind of tea leaves that is demanded. For old and thick tea leaves, the roasting time needs to be shortened. The tenderness of the tea leaves needs a higher temperature when compared to the old ones, the process of roasting begins from a medium to a high temperature. The temperature is between 90 and 100°C and is roasted for 4 to 10 hours. After this, the temperature has to be reduced to 80-85 °C for a period of 2 to 4 hours. This process is used to make sure that the drink has a good taste without acrimony and keeps back the character and fragrance of the tea leaves.

Shape and tightness

The tea leaves that have a tight shape are kind of more resistant to heat. The temperature during roasting must be reduced to 85-90 °C and with longer hours. As for the tea leaves that are loose, the right temperature for roasting must be 100 °C and for a short period.

Aromas

The smell of the oolong tea is one of the things that makes this tea so special. Nevertheless, it's one of the most difficult to regulate. The difference in the processing has the tendency of having an impact on the aroma of the tea. The outcome will be extremely volatile. Mild aromas can certainly evaporate during the process of roasting when the baking and temperature time isn't properly controlled.

Below is a list of the different fire levels and their equivalent scent that the farmer desires to get at the end of his processing.

- **Low fire**: This is wonderful if you want to derive a flowery scent. The outcome of the tea in this level will steep a light yellow liquor. The appearance of the leaves after steeping is green with read.
- **Medium fire**: This is an idea for leaves that can give out a fruity scent. Gold yellow will be the color of the liquor.
- **High fire**: The end result is a scent that is like caramel. The color of the liquor could be orange or dark yellow.

Normally, it is advised that lower temperature and a shorter roasting time should be used for teas with good quality and fresh scents. Tea that has lower quality and less fragrance, it is suggested to use long roasting time and high temperature to supersede the lack of quality. In the latter case, the best will be made out of the tea by the tea master. The urgencies are to lower the content of water and remove the smell that wasn't having a pleasant scent. Finally, it is necessary to bring to your notice that the consumer's demand for the tea will be dependent on the level of roasting. It is normally known that the tea drinks from Guangdong do prefer a darker roast than other parts of China.

On a brighter note, to maintain the strong aroma and green color of the tea, the temperature has between 60 °C - 70 °C and the time will be regulated until the content of the water go up from 5% to 6%.

Flavors

Peradventure the tea leaves are mellow in flavor and sweet, they must be roasted with a temperature of 80-85 °C for a period of 4 to 6 hours, while for temperature between 75-80 °C, the time period should be 2 to 3 hours the subsequent day. The avoidance of high temperature can help in preventing the tea from tasting bitter or rip and at the end maintain the tea quality.

Heat Control

The heat control spells the changes in the appearance and the level of chemical to the tea leaves in the process of roasting. This affects the shape of the tea leaves in color and brewing after. The color during the brewing process is also changed. The right heat control can supplement the insufficiency of the tea quality. The improper control will lower the quality. For some types unique teas, once the heat is correctly controlled, the nuances in flavor and aroma. There are different kinds of tea and their heat resistance level all differ.

The Oolong Tea Recipes

Traditional Thai Iced Tea Recipe Cha Yen from Thailand

The tea is called Cha Yen in Thailand and it translates to Tea cool or chilled tea. So for this section, we will look at one of the recipes of oolong tea.

Things needed:

- 1 can of Evaporated Milk
- 6 cups of Water
- 1 cup of oolong tea (Thai Tea)
- 1 cup of sugar
- Half-and-Half Cream (a western touch)

Procedures:

- Take the water and put it in a large pan or pot and set on fire.

- You can now add the tea and take off the saucepan from the fire

- Then you should stir to immerse all the leaves in the tea into the water.

You should then steep the leaves for about 5 minutes.

1. Dispense the drink through a coffee sieve or a well-meshed filter into a large jug.

2. Add the sugar to the hot tea and mix continually in order to liquefy.

3. Cool it to room temperature.

4. Close and refrigerate until you are ready to serve.

5. Then you should fill the cup to use with crushed ice. The cup should be tall

6. Add sufficient amount of the tea to fill the cup to reach up to 1 inch from the top of the cup.

7. Put 3 to 4 tablespoons of the evaporated milk into the ice in each cup.

8. Finally, to have a good and lovely taste, you can add the half creamer with the evaporated milk or rather the evaporated milk only

Bubble Tea Sugar Syrup

Ingredient needed:

- 1 cup of brown sugar
- 1 cup of white sugar
- 2 cups water
- 1 cup of oolong tea.

Procedures:

- Firstly, mix the water, tea, and sugar in a larger pot

- Secondly, cook the mixture of water and sugar in a fire that is either high or medium heat

- Immediately the mixture has boiled, take it down from your source of heat

- Allow it to cool and you can now enjoy it. You can refrigerate the excess for later consumption

Why Oolong Tea?

Listed as part of the most recognized type of tea in Taiwan and China, it is regarded to have a lot of health benefits when it is taken on a regular basis. It is loaded with antioxidants, caffeine helps in fighting free radicals and the leaf itself has catechin. It is used for different purposes because of its healing properties that it possess and can be seen in many grocery stores. So here are some of the benefits of this wonderful plant

CHAPTER SEVEN

General Benefits of Oolong Tea

1. It boosts your metabolism leading to weight loss.

It aids in the burning of fat quickly through the raising up of the metabolism process for two hours after it has been drank. It has polyphenols in it, which aids in the blocking of enzymes that build fat. This connotes that while you take oolong tea, you can lose weight. This is possible if you don't add it with artificial sweeteners or sugar. Peradventure, you want something sweet, then you should consider the addition of a littler raw honey, stevia, maple syrup or agave syrup, which all have low sugar on the glycemic index.

2. Lowers cholesterol

The oolong tea has been recognized to help in the reduction of the cholesterol levels and improve the health of the heart. The tea is semi-oxidized, it manufacturers a good amount of polyphenol molecules, which has the ability to trigger the enzyme lipase. This is known to help in the dissolving of fat in the body

3. Increases mental alertness

Taking oolong tea helps in the revitalization of your performance and mental alertness, this is so because of the caffeine content in it. Sensitive to caffeine? Then you should be very careful and have a limitation to how you consume it.

4. Aids digestion

The tea supports actively in the digestion process mostly for people who aren't sensitive to caffeine. What it does, is to alkalized the digestive tracts, and help in the reduction of inflammation for those who have ulcer problems of acid reflux. Due to its mildly antiseptic, it has the capacity of removing bacteria from the stomach. It is calm and has a smooth flavor which aids in the soothing of the stomach when it is consumed hot

5. Promotes healthy hair

Because of the high antioxidants level in it, the oolong tea can help in the prevention of the loss of hair. It can also make your hair to be shinier and thicker.

6. Betters your skin condition

Sensitivities or allergies do occur in conjunction with eczema. The oolong tea has the ability to suppress the allergic reactions that should have taken place because it helps in the combating of the free radicals, this is part of the healing qualities of an antioxidant. Apart from this, the antioxidant that is found in the leaves of the oolong is important for a skin that is vibrant and young. Aging process can be slowed down rapidly by simply drinking the oolong tea. It's a wonderful tool for the anti-aging process

7. Stabilizes blood sugar

For those that have diabetes type 2, you can elevate the blood glucose levels when you take oolong tea. Different studies have demonstrated how who are suffering from diabetes can greatly benefit through the drinking of the oolong tea. According to the studies carried out, it decreases the blood glucose to a more healthy level. The antioxidants that are in the oolong leave is gotten from the polyphenols, this does wonder in the metabolizing of sugar

8. Prevents tooth decay

The green and oolong tea helps in the protection of the teeth from acids that are manufactured by some bacteria. The manufacturing of this acid and the development of the growth are subdued when you drink the oolong tea, which signifies that it is efficient in the reducing or preventing the decay of the tooth and build up the plaque.

9. Prevents osteoporosis and forms strong bones

The oolong tea can help in the preventing of osteoporosis and protect your bones. For those who drink the oolong tea consistently, are more likely to give off some bone mineral density, aid in the retention of minerals from healthy food eaten. The oolong tea has been discovered to have calcium and magnesium in its leaves.

10. Strengthens the immune system

Apart from all these benefits, it is well-known for the anti-cancer ability. The tea supports the maintenance of a good and vibrant immune system. The tea has the antioxidant flavonoids and helps in stopping cellular damage.

Oolong Tea Benefits for Skin:

The frequent consumption of the oolong tea does excellently good works on the skin. A large number of problems that have to do with the skin is caused by the exposure of free radicals. Well, you need not worry because it has polyphenols which kill the radicals then give off stress from a range of different skin problems. Apart from the general benefits discussed above, the following are specific benefit you will derive from the consumption of the oolong tea intended for your skin

- **Treatment of Eczema (known as Atopic Dermatitis)**

Eczema, which is also known as atopic dermatitis is a prolonged skin infection or disease which can be characterized by redness, itching, scarring, swelling and most times infections of the lesion as a result of the continuous scratching. Studies have exposed that people who mix the dermatological cure for this situation in line with the intake of a minimum of 3 tea cup of the oolong tea per day, do experience more liberation when compared to patients who don't consume the tea at all.

- **The benefit of Anti-aging:**

The frequent disclosure of the skin to the free radicals speeds up the procedure of getting old and lower the rate at which exfoliation takes place, this will result in the immature occurrence of dark spots or and wrinkles on the skin. But because of the level of antioxidants, which is high in it, the tea rather decreases the rust of the body cells, resulting in a much healthy looking skin.

- **Improves the vitality of your Skin:**

The frequent intake of the oolong tea helps in the reduction of wrinkles and help in the improvement of the elasticity and toning of the skin, thereby giving you that youthful look or appearance. The skin is protected by the polyphenols that are available in it and stop it from any destruction as a result of disclosure to the sun.

The Hair Benefits of Oolong Tea

These benefits have only come to the knowledge of many recently and has been one of the most used ingredients in quite a quantity of hair maintenance products. The tea can be likened to an herbal fermentation, which is made from the tender portions of the plant such as leaves, shoots, and flowers. This promotes the development of a good and healthy hair. The benefits that can be derived when used in the circumstance of the maintenance of the hair, are listed below.

- **Prevention of the loss of Hair:**

The presence of the antioxidants in the oolong tea is widely known to certify the proper breakdown of the hormone in male. The changes in the DHT during its metabolic action give rise to a hair loss. So do a tea and rinse it with the leaves will be of immense benefit in the prevention of the extreme peeling of the hair.

- **Promotes a shiny and Healthy Hair:**

The tea that is made from the leaves of the oolong has a pleasant nature and is mild. It didn't only make the hair to be soft, but makes it look shiny.

Weight Loss Benefit of The Oolong Tea

- Due to the rich content of the antioxidants in it, it helps in the enhancement of the metabolism process by 10 percent for some hours after the intake of the oolong tea and also aid in the protection from different chronic diseases.

- The antioxidant helps in blazing fat faster and more efficiently, which helps in losing weight and gives a healthy functionality in the immune system.

- The caffeine content in it helps in the fat oxidation process

- It controls the blood sugar level and lowers the cravings for more sugar

- It helps in maximizing the power of the body.

- Taking oolong tea helps in the prevention of obesity

Nutritional Value of Oolong Tea

The oolong tea has a rich content of antioxidants. The following are some of the various minerals that it contains, calcium, potassium, copper, manganese, selenium, carotene besides vitamins A, C, E, B and K. adding to these minerals, it also contains niacinamide, folic acid and extra purifying alkaloids that you haven't thought about. As a result of its semi-fermented feature, the oolong tea also contains a lot of polyphenolic elements, which give off an additional benefits health wise. Like all others, the tea leaves do contain some amount of caffeine. During the process of the making of the oolong tea, the tea decreases the content of the caffeine significantly.

How Much Quantity Should I Take?

After boiling your water, add a cup of the oolong tea, this could be in the teabag form or using tablespoon from the loose leaves. Keep for a maximum of 4 minutes and take it when it is still hot and you will surely enjoy it. It's necessary for you to take the oolong tea in balance or moderation due to it caffeine quantity. Taking too much of this oolong tea, which has caffeine has some side effects which include, irregular heartbeat, headaches, inflammation, irritable bowel syndrome, and anxiety. For those who are breastfeeding, pregnant or do have serious medical challenges, which is affected by the consumption of caffeine, must first talk to their doctor before taking it. As they normally say, prevention is better than cure.

Before The Consumption of Oolong Tea, Think of This

It is evident that the oolong tea does perform wonders from the benefits listed in this book. Conversely, it is important for you to take some precaution and take it in control. As stated earlier, the tea has some quantity of caffeine, the consumption of it too much has its own side effects. Nobody wants to take something that will have a negative effect on their body. The side effects range from an irregular heartbeat, heartburn, irritable bowel syndrome, minor to severe headaches, vomiting, and nervousness. These are just a few to mention from the many side effects. It has been advised that women who are pregnant should keep tag on the cup of tea that is taken daily. Consumption of it daily will make the caffeine to hurt the baby. So keep this point in your thought and go forward and have a wonderful time taking oolong tea. Have a "cuppa!" experience.

Bottom Line for Oolong Tea

The leaves are rolled or curled into a crispy shape, which has the resemblance of a tiny black dragon, therefore this is the reason behind the description of its name. They are usually harvested late in the spring when compared to white teas or green tea and are more mature. White tea or green teas are usually harvested late April or early May. The manufacturing of the oolong tea is kind of complicated because some steps are repeated different times before the final browning a bruising of the leaves is gotten. Withering, firing, shaping and rolling are similar to the black tea, but the only difference is that much temperature and attention to accurate timing is required or necessary.

CHAPTER EIGHT

The Wonders of Black Tea

B lack tea is a unique kind of tea. It is inherently more oxidized than the green tea, white tea, and oolong tea and possesses a kind of flavor that is a whole lot stronger than each of the other teas. Black tea is made from the leaves of a shrub, called *Camellia sinensis*. The plant occurs in two different varieties (i.e., the small-leaved and large-leaved plants) and both are utilized for the production of black tea.

Unlike green tea that easily loses its flavor within one year, black tea actually retains its flavor for lots of years. This feature makes it particularly easy to trade, without having to worry about spoilage or reduction in quality. As a matter of fact, this unique feature of black tea also made it to be compressed into brick forms and utilized as some sort of currency, in Siberia, Tibet, and Mongolia, at the start of the 19th century. At the present, rather unsurprisingly, black tea actually accounts for more than 90% of all the tea currently sold in the western regions.

History of Black Tea in China

It is practically impossible to discuss black tea without mentioning China. When it comes to "all things tea," China is always a reference point. All other locations and producers are merely offshoots of the production and procedures that originated in ancient China. In China's local mandarin, it's known as "red tea," due to its reddish-black characteristic color.

In China, prior to the late 16th century, the common tea types were the Oolong (also called semi-oxidized) and green (completely unoxidized) teas. Oxidation here simply means how much exposure to oxygen (air) it has, after harvest. Like most remarkable discoveries of the world, the black tea came into existence by accident. Around 1590, stories have it that, a passing army reached the Fujian province and decided to have some rest at a close-by tea factory. As expected, the production process needed to be suspended, to afford the soldiers all the room they need. While this was going on, the collected tea leaves that were left out in the sun (probably for partial oxidation), stayed out there, a little longer than usual and this made the leaves to turn black, due to the extended period of oxidation it had witnessed. Upon the departure of the soldiers, production resumed again, but this time, it was not to brew the green tea or oolong tea, but the very first set of black teas. The tea was then named Lapsang Souchong after the name of the mountainous are (Lapsang) and the tea plant (Souchong).

They are many variations in the black tea production process, hence different types of black teas often result. Some of the common ones are Fujian Minhong, Fujian Lapsang Souchong, Anhui Keemun, Guangdong Yingteh, Sichuan Mabian Gongfu and Yunnan Dianhong black teas. Out of all these though, the Keemun black tea is usually the commonest.

Keemun Black Tea

This tea was produced for the first time around 1875 by Hu Yuanlong in the Qimen County. Yuanlong was actually on a trip to Fujian with the mission of improving his skills as a tea maker (talk about loving your job!) Upon his return from Fujian, he began to brew his own tea locally in Qimen, customizing the entire process and making it his personal signature. Not too long after that, his customers observed that the tea was so unique, that they patronized him more and more. That tea eventually was known as the Keemun black tea and before you know it, the fame of that tea has spread across all China like wildfire and it soon became the most desired tea in all of China. Indeed, diligence pays off, this Hu Yuanlong teaches us very clearly.

In China, the Keemun black tea (and all the other black teas) are taken "black," but in the western world, this may not always be so. Most western people love to add a mixture of milk and some sugar, while some others prefer to use just honey, to enhance the taste and the fragrance of the tea. Irrespective of the additives, the Keemun black tea still remains an excellent choice, in terms of nutrition and aroma.

History of Black Tea in Europe

The history of the black tea in European countries can actually be traced all the way back to the 17th century, when explorers from Europe, found themselves in China. As expected, you could not possibly visit China during this period and not have a taste of some good tea. When these explorers tasted the tea and just could not have enough of it, they decided to take it along with them to Europe. So, the first real record of black tea in Europe took place around 1610. This was also facilitated by the Dutch merchants who brought the tea in large quantities from China and carried out the distribution in Europe.

This tea was so highly valued upon its initial introduction to England and was regarded as a "mysterious oriental drink." Of course, it commanded very high prices, which only the wealthy could afford. Soon, the drink became a symbol of wealth and a show of class. And when anybody really wants to throw a truly remarkable party, he served tea, to his guests.

History of Black Tea in England

England is particularly renowned for tea. The British have so much passion about tea in so much that it's almost impossible to imagine the British without tea. History has it that in 1662, when King Charles was to marry the Portuguese princess, Catherine, the princess brought lots of black tea crates to the king, as a form of dowry. This action gave birth to black tea in the palace of the king. The consumption of this tea began to grow in the king's palace in so much that the tradition soon spread to the common people. Now it is basically an impossibility to imagine the queen or any other royalty, without tea. As a matter of fact, information has it that when the British Queen wakes up every day, the first thing she does is to take a nice and hot cup of tea.

In the year 1840, Anna Telford, (the Duchess at the time) brought about the concept of afternoon tea. At this time, the price of tea was already coming down (not that it matters to her) so it was more affordable. They could now take tea in the morning and afternoon, while they use the opportunity to trade the latest gossips.

Now, tea breaks and coffee breaks have become a tradition, not restricted to England alone, but even America and many parts of the world.

Production Process of Black Tea

There are various steps involved in the production of good black tea. The major steps are discussed below:

1. **Harvest of the Leaves:** Of course, this is the first step in the production of any plant based product. *Camellia sinensis* is a shrub (about 1 meter tall), so the harvesting of the leaves is always a very easy

process. The harvesting may be done manually or mechanically, depending on the orientation of the farm and available resources.

2. **Withering of the leaves:** The withering process is carried out, basically to remove some water from the harvested leaves. This process is usually done by blowing air on the leaves, either in a natural environment or specialized air blowers (large scale production).

3. **Processing of the withered leaves:** There are two principal methods of processing the withered leaves. These are the Orthodox and the CTC (Crush, Tear, and Curl) methods.

- **Orthodox method:** This type of processing can be done by hand or with machines such as a rotovane or cylindrical rolling table. Usually, the hand processing is utilized for teas of very high quality. In the leaf processing, the tea leaves are rolled heavily either with the hand or mechanically and this produces a blend of broken leaves as well as whole leaves, which are subsequently sorted from each other and allowed to fully oxidize before finally drying. The important thing to note in this method is that the leaves produced after this process, have relatively large particle sizes and some can even remain as whole leaves. So, the leaves that result here are best utilized by those who intend to prepare the leaves for some kind of "concussion" and then manually sieve off the leaves afterward.

- **CTC method:** The "cut, tear and curl" method is a technique used in producing fine or dust-grade leaves which are utilized in making tea bags. The method was invented in 1930 by William McKercher. This method is considered by most people as a significant improvement on the orthodox method, in the production of black tea. After leaves are passed through the rotovane (which breaks it into smaller fragments), the broken leaves are then passed into the CTC machine, which completes the process of shredding and crushing into very fine particles. As expected this is the method used by large scale producers of black tea.

4. **Oxidation or Fermentation:** After the fragmenting or crushing of the leaves, they are then oxidized in a climate controlled environment. The word "fermentation" may be misleading because no actual fermentation occurs in the process. This process is very key to the production of black tea because the amount/level of oxidation is what determines the eventual color of the tea. So, to produce black tea, the fragmented or crushed leaves are allowed to oxidize for a long time. This enables its color to change to black. Conversely, to produce Oolong tea, the amount of oxidation here will be a partial one and to produce green tea, no oxidation will be witnessed at this stage.

5. **Drying of the leaves:** Once the desired level of oxidation has been attained, the process is "arrested," by drying the leaves. So, the level of oxidation attained here is all that will remain with the leaves, until consumption.

6. **Sorting and Packaging:** Once the drying process is complete, the dried leaves are then graded and separated, depending on the particle sizes. After sorting, they are then packaged into the required materials and moved for supply or consumption.

General Health Benefits of Black Tea

It is always a great idea to incorporate black tea into your diet because it comes with tons of health benefits and this is natural because it contains an amazingly balanced nutrient profile. The increase in oxidation process allows it to contain higher levels of caffeine and flavor than the other tea types.

Some of the numerous health benefits of black tea are given below:

1. **Cardiovascular Benefits:** From numerous research, it has been established that the consumption of black tea actually reduces the risk of coming down with cardiovascular diseases. Black tea contains anti-oxidants which play an important role in preventing the oxidation of LDL (Low-Density Lipoprotein) cholesterol. This also helps in protecting the walls of the arteries and reduces the risk of heart diseases. As

a matter of fact, black tea consumption has been found to completely reverse some coronary heart diseases. So, long story short, black tea helps protect your heart.

2. **Prevention of Cancer:** Black tea contains polyphenols, which are antioxidants. These polyphenols help in preventing the formation of carcinogenic substances in the body system, hence, considerably reducing the risk of coming down with some cancers. In fact, from research, it has been established that black tea actually helps to prevent breast and prostate cancer.

3. **Elimination of Free Radicals:** In simple terms, free radicals are the by-products of most of our digestion processes. Free radicals become particularly prominent in our body systems when we indulge ourselves in unhealthy foods. The downside of these free radicals is that they can actually cause a lot of complications in the body such as cancer and atherosclerosis (narrowing and hardening of the blood vessels). The good news is that black tea is actually fortified with a lot of antioxidants, which easily get rid of these free radicals and clean up the body system, hence reducing the risk of coming down with some of these ailments.

4. **Enhancement of the Immune System:** The Immune system is basically our principal line of defense against illnesses and diseases, caused by different pathogens such as bacteria and viruses. Black tea

contains tannins which have to capability to actively ward off these pathogens along with their infections, hence improving the efficiency of the immune system and allowing for a better overall state of health.

5. **Improvement of the Oral Health:** Black tea contains catechin antioxidants that play a vital role in reducing the appearance of oral cancers. Also, the tannins and polyphenols it contains, also acts as potent antibiotics, thereby inhibiting the growth of bacteria that cause tooth decay.

6. **Enhancement of the Brain and Nervous System:** Black tea contains caffeine which (in moderate quantity) enhances the blood flow inside the brain. Though excessively high caffeine levels can also be harmful, black tea contains just the right amount of it to keep the brain functioning properly, unlike coffee which can contain excessively high levels sometimes. Black tea also enhances concentration and mental alertness, thus allowing you to easily pay maximum attention and concentration to any assignment you are carrying out. Also, from research, regular consumption of black tea has been shown to protect against Parkinson's disease.

7. **Enhancement of Digestive Tract Functioning:** The tannins present in black tea have therapeutic effects on the gastro-intestinal tract and help to ward off intestinal illnesses.

8. **Enhancement of Healthy Bone Formation:** Black tea helps to greatly reduce the risk of osteoporosis (poor bone formation), due to the different phytochemicals it possesses. So, generally, people who take black tea regularly, tend to develop healthier bones.

9. **Easy Source of Energy:** The presence of caffeine makes black tea to be considered as a major energy drink. This stimulant heightens the alertness level of the brain and muscles (hence making them energized). As a matter of fact, though the quantity of caffeine in black tea is less than that of coffee, it actually has a more stimulating effect than coffee.

10. **Enhances weight loss:** Black tea is particularly recommended for those who are looking to lose some weight, due to its low level of fat, sodium, and calories. So, this makes it far superior to unhealthy drinks such as soda or other beverages with high fat and sodium content. In addition, black tea also enhances the activity of the metabolic process, hence also contributing to loss of weight.

11. **Reduction of Cholesterol level:** Bad cholesterol is the fear of many people and the major reason they don't eat a lot of foods. Black tea actually possesses the ability to reduce the triglyceride levels in the body, thus the incidence of bad cholesterol is greatly reduced and by extension, the risk of having a heart disease is greatly reduced as well. Drinking a few cups of black tea on daily basis, prevents the

formation of plaques (clogs) inside the arteries, hence preventing the incidence of hypertension of heart failure.

12. **Relief for Stress:** Though this may seem psychological, it also has a touch of physiological changes in it. Stress builds up when we engage in strenuous activities (which are often necessary) and when this happens, the muscles get weaker and require a means of regaining the expended energy and this is why you feel tired. A cup of black tea often gets the job done in most cases, as it contains L-theanine which enhances stress relief. So, after a long, hard, day, a cup of black tea (hot or cold) is always a good idea.

How to Prepare a Delicious Cup of Black Tea

Most people don't get the best out of their black tea, simply because they really don't know how to prepare it properly. Generally, for maximum enjoyment of your black tea, there are a few specifications you must follow. The first thing is a hot cup of water (preferably boiling). One teaspoonful of tea should go into about 200ml of hot water, stirred and allowed to stay for about 60 seconds. Higher quantities of water will basically just make the taste of the tea to be lost. For some special black teas like Darjeeling, the tea should be allowed to stay in the water for about 3-4 minutes before sieving or removal of the teabag. And there you go! Your delicious tea is ready to drink.

Note of Caution While Taking Black Tea

There's a common saying that goes thus; "when the purpose of a thing is not known, abuse is inevitable." Substance abuse nowadays is considered a criminal offense. But did you know that cocaine or heroin, do not necessarily have to be evil? They could be put to good use, but some "tough guy" would just prefer to abuse it.

The story is similar for tea. Though it has tons of benefits and seems like the perfect health drink, overtaking it (as much as 5-10 cups per day), can result in serious side effects and complications. These side effects are principally due to its caffeine content which is a Central Nervous System (CNS) stimulant. So, if the CNS is "over-stimulated," some complications can result. Some of these complications include:

- Diarrhea
- Vomiting
- Irritability
- Tremor
- Irregular heartbeat
- Dizziness
- Heartburn
- Ringing ears and
- Convulsions.

No matter how much you love black tea, if you are pregnant or lactating, you should not take more than 2 cups per day. On a general level, 2-3 cups of black tea are the recommended amount per day.

CHAPTER NINE

Benefits of Black Tea for the Skin

B lack tea doesn't just come with a variety of health benefits alone, it also comes with a wide range of advantages for your skin care. Many constituents of black tea, such as vitamins E, C, and B2, as well as minerals like potassium, magnesium, and zinc, making it a very good option for skin care and protection. Some of the specific details of this are discussed below:

1. **Prevention of skin infections:** The high caffeine content of black teas, doesn't just enhance alertness, it also helps in killing oral viruses, thus preventing infection of the skin and giving you a generally blemish-free skin.

2. **Reduction of eye puffiness:** Did you know that even after extracting the tea from the tea bag (after immersion), the teabag is not useless? You can actually place them on your eyelids (especially after

enduring sleepless nights because of exams) and watch as the puffed eyes magically return to normal.

3. **Prevention of Pimples:** I can bet you that nobody loves to have pimples! They can be so annoying. The good news is; with a cup (or two) of black tea daily, you can as well forget about having pimples. Black tea also helps in preventing premature aging and wrinkles.

4. **Prevention of skin cancer:** This is another very important feature of the black tea. The presence of antioxidants actually helps in significantly reducing the incidence of skin cancer.

5. **Skin protection:** Black tea can actually be very effective as a sun blocking agent when the extract is rubbed on the skin.

6. **Skin regeneration:** This feature is facilitated by the presence of tannins and polyphenols present in the black tea. These compounds enhance cell regeneration and by extension, skin regeneration.

7. **Contribution to a glowing skin:** The tannins play an important role in protecting the skin from harmful environmental impacts, thus allowing the skin to remain radiant and blemish-free. It also enhances the circulation of blood, which also helps to maintain the health of the skin.

How to Use Tea to Clear Your Skin

It is no news that we live in an age of global warming where pollutants are all around us 24 hours a day. Some of these pollutants can settle on the skin and cause some serious complications. We may not be able to stop the globe from "warming up," but we can, at last, protect ourselves from its deleterious effect without breaking the bank in the process; all with the help of tea.

It is also no news that tea is actually an excellent health drink and you may probably even be aware that it has an amazing effect on skin care, but what you may not know is that there are many ways of utilizing tea for skin protection and care. Some of these ways are as follows:

1. **Drinking it:** This is perhaps the commonest use of tea to most people and it's only natural because hunger and thirst are a basic biological instinct which must regularly be satisfied. Drinking tea does your skin a world of good (as discussed earlier) because of its different unique constituents. While planning to drink your tea though, you may want to consider squeezing some lemon in it. This allows for better digestion and assimilation.

2. **By topical application:** Topical application simply means rubbing it on your skin. This is pretty simple actually; once you've brewed your fresh cup of tea, instead of drinking it, just get some cotton ball, dip it in the tea and rub it on your skin. Another effective

variation to this technique is to, first of all, freeze the tea and then slide the ice cube over your skin. Believe me, this can be so awesome especially on hot days!

3. **Addition to beauty products:** Tea can also be added to your beauty products. A few tablespoons of brewed tea can be added to your lotion, you can then apply it on your skin, the same way you always have; the only difference now is that your lotion now has an upgrade. Apart from keeping your skin smooth and fresh, tea also has "sun-screen" capabilities, protecting you from the harsh radiation on sunny days.

4. **Make a toner with it:** Tea possesses anti-bacterial and pH balancing properties and this makes it an excellent candidate for the production of toners. Instead of wasting your hard-earned money on expensive toners that are chemically synthesized, you could produce your very own "all-natural" toner, with a few simple ingredients that are easy to get. All you need is 1/4 c of your freshly brewed black tea, together with about 3 tablespoons of your organic apple cider vinegar. Then pour the mixture in about 1/4 c of water and shake it up! There you have it! Your very own homemade toner. You can simply apply it every morning or late at night before going to bed.

5. **Steam it:** Steaming is perhaps one method of tea utilization many are unfamiliar with. Some may even think; does that work? Oh, I can assure you, it definitely does. In case you don't know, the skin is

actually the largest organ in the human body and it possesses the capability to absorb nutrients. This is because it possesses pore spaces through which it "breathes." Steaming your black tea is a relatively easy process:

- Brew your black tea in a hot, boiling water placed on your gas or electric burner

- When the steam begins to emerge, reduce the heat from your burner to allow for a constant steam

- Place your face in the steam, breathe it in and relax

- After some minutes, clean the accumulated sweat off your face and repeat the process

- Once you've done this for about 10 minutes, your skin is sure to have obtained the maximum benefits from the process, so, you can clean up your face with warm water or even go for a shower.

Benefits of Face-Steaming with Black Tea

Before we go into the benefits of face steaming, there are a few things you should probably know. Firstly, you should know that the skin can be very absorbent (and this can be both good and bad). When you sweat, if proper hygiene is not maintained, the dirt begins to "clog-up" in your face pores and this begins to cause spots on your face. When these spots successfully form and dry-up though, they become quite difficult to get out. this is where steaming your face with black tea comes in.

The principal benefit of face steaming is that substances trapped in your face pores actually get purged out when you steam your face and this gives you a healthier, fresher and better-looking skin. Your skin can now "breathe" normally once again and you will equally feel fresher and more alive. In summary, the remarkable benefits of face steaming with black tea are as follows:

- **Increased blood circulation to your face:** When you steam your face with black tea, your face gets an increased flow of blood. The benefits of this are actually numerous, but the principal one is that your skin gets more oxygen and nutrient supply and this allows for maximum skin functioning and inevitably; an incredibly radiant glow!

- **Increased level of perspiration:** When you steam your face, there is an outflow of toxins and dead cells and this plays no small role, in maintaining a healthy skin.

- **Unclogging of pores:** Steaming of the face allows the hardened oils (on the face) to soften-up, hence making them very easy to remove

- **Maintenance of youthful skin:** Face steaming moisturizes your skin like no moisturizer can! This is particularly good because skin moisturization plays a key role in preventing aging of the skin cells. So, you can keep looking young and fresh every day, even if you're in your fifties.

- **Acne prevention and treatment:** The heat from the steam and the anti-microbial properties of Tea ensure that any bacteria present on your face get killed whenever you do a black tea face steaming.

How to Make Face Masks with Black Tea

Face masks can be very remarkable! This is principal because it affords the "mask ingredients" direct contact with the face, which allows for direct action on the skin. If you are looking to get rid of those emerging wrinkles or acne on your face, then you might want to consider a face mask.

Black tea face masks are particularly great because of the numerous health properties embedded in black tea. There are various recipes that can be used to make face masks, with black tea as the active ingredient and these ingredients are very easy (and cheap) to get. Though there are many different combinations of recipes, I've found this one combination to be particularly healthy and effective; this involves the use of black tea, honey and real lemon juice.

Black tea, honey, and lemon juice mask: All you need to make this face mask is just 1 teaspoon of lemon juice (freshly squeezed), 1 tablespoon of honey, 3 black-tea bags and about a quarter-filled cup of hot water. Firstly, place the tea bags in the cup of hot water and allow it steep for 2-3 minutes. After this, drain the water and press the tea bags to ensure most of the water is out. After this, cut open the tea bags into a small cup or container, add the tablespoon of honey and the teaspoon of lemon juice and stir together with a spoon. Once this is done, then you are now ready to apply the mixture on your face. Use your hand (it's simple and works fine) to apply the mixture on your face, but avoid covering your eyelids, to prevent seepage into your eyes. Leave on the mask on your face for about 5 minutes and then gently massage your face (with the mask on) to exfoliate your skin. After this, you can then wash off the mask with some warm water. If your skin is naturally dry, you can apply your moisturizer afterward and watch yourself radiate and glow!

These recipes are particularly excellent for the following reasons:

- **Black tea** contains tannins and polyphenols that enhance skin regeneration and pimple prevention, not to mention the ameliorating effect of caffeine on eye puffiness. These properties among others, make the black tea an essential ingredient in making your face mask.

- **Honey** naturally possesses antibacterial properties, making it an excellent treatment for acne. So, basically, if your major motivation for making a face mask is because of acne, then honey is one ingredient you definitely cannot afford to leave out. Apart from being an excellent treatment for acne, it contains loads of antioxidants which function greatly in slowing down the aging process. In addition to that, it possesses really fantastic moisturizing properties, which makes you to naturally glow!

- **Lemon juice** equally shares many of the remarkable properties of honey. It comes with antibacterial properties that help in the prevention and treatment of various levels of blemishes. Another unique feature of the lemon juice is that it actually helps in the treatment of scars. So, if you happen to have some spots or scars on your face that you would really love to get rid of, then you might want to seriously consider adding the lemon juice into your next face mask. Lemon possesses citric acid, which is actually very effective in the removal of the top (discolored) layers of dying or dead layers of the skin. This inevitably leaves your skin smooth, fresh and radiant, helping you re-live your teenage years all over again (only this time, you're way cooler and more experienced than you were back then!)

Bottom Line for Black Tea

Black tea is indeed a wonder! It comes with so many amazing benefits that allow for proper functioning of the body organs. If you fall in the "beer and soda" family, you need to seriously reconsider your preferences in drinks and switch to the more healthy, natural and refreshing black tea. If you are the type that loves "sweet stuff," you can as well add as much honey or sugar as you like, to complement that excellent cup of healthy drink. Black tea is too great a drink for anyone to miss out, not to mention the numerous application methods, to benefit the skin. If you haven't done so already, get a pack or two of this healthy black tea, on your next grocery shopping and you will be glad you did.

About the Author

L aura Victoria is a level 2 & 3 trained beauty therapist specializing in skin care, including aesthetics.

Trained in Harley street, London, she understands the needs of skin and how to get the best results using natural tea products, including the amazing benefits of using tea not just for internal health but the benefits of tea as skincare.

She owns her own clinic, Therabeautique, based in south east London.

Book Outline

In this book you will learn and discover how tea can benefit and improve your skin, this book will cover green tea, white tea, black tea and Oolong tea will help renew your skin with that glow from within look.

Learn recipes and tricks to get the best results and the secrets to great skin!

www.ingramcontent.com/pod-product-compliance
Lightning Source LLC
Chambersburg PA
CBHW062014280526
45787CB00005B/2097